EVALUATION OF JOINT MOTION

Evaluation of Joint Motion: Methods of Measurement and Recording

by Dortha Esch and Marvin Lepley

Illustrations by Jean Magney

University of Minnesota Press
Minneapolis

Published by the University of Minnesota Press
111 Third Avenue South, Suite 290, Minneapolis, MN 55401-2520

Printed in the United States of America at
the University of Minnesota Printing Department.
Eighth printing, 1997

Library of Congress Catalog Card Number: 73-93576
ISBN 0-8166-0714-1

Preface

The measurement of the motion produced by an individual in any given joint of the body is done to determine the degree and extent of loss of mobility resulting from injury, disease, or disuse. The record obtained from such measurement provides a basis for patient treatment planning by therapists, nurses, physicians, and other members of the health care team.

The techniques of measurement and the methods of recording are not difficult to learn. To ensure proper patient care each member of the health care team, even if he is not required to evaluate and record, should have an appreciation of the problems faced by a person with joint impairment. Such an understanding is enhanced by studying the techniques of measuring joint motion.

This manual presents the most commonly accepted methods of measurement, the full-circle or 360° system and the half-circle or 180° system. A special unit on hand evaluation by use of graphic means is included.

This manual has been used in the classroom for several years previous to publication. We have found that students learn measurement techniques and recording with ease because each page following the introductory material provides a guide to the technique for measuring a joint of the body. Directions for the testing position and placement of the measuring instrument are given. Illustrations show graphically correct instrument placement and give the normal limits of motion for each joint. A form is provided to record the measurements obtained. Students are able to study the manual quite independently and learn techniques with minimal instructor assistance.

Since there is considerable variability in normal limits of motion figures given by various authors, we have arbitrarily selected one set: those used by the Physical Medicine Department of the University of Minnesota with some modifications resulting from our own observations in the clinic and classroom.

It is our belief that the manual presents a practical approach to learning and may be successfully used by students, therapists, and others who are required to evaluate joint mobility.

We would like to express appreciation to all our colleagues who have willingly consulted with us during the preparation of this manual. We especially want to thank John D. Allison, R.P.T., and James F. Pohtilla, R.P.T., who provided information and valuable suggestions during the early development of the manual. Special thanks go to Darlene Kriska and Barbara Bartholomew who typed the manuscript. Their pleasant and cooperative attitude was appreciated.

The preparation of the manual was assisted financially, in part, by S.R.S. Grant No. 16-P-56810, awarded to the Regional Rehabilitation Research and Training Center, RT-2, at the University of Minnesota Medical School.

Dortha Esch, B.S., O.T.R.
Marvin Lepley, B.S., O.T.R.

University of Minnesota
October 1973

Contents

EVALUATION OF JOINT MOTION

Introduction

The measurement of joint motion is one of a number of evaluative procedures important in programs for rehabilitation of the physically handicapped. Effective rehabilitation planning requires consideration of all aspects of behavior, including the degree to which an individual can move, for this influences the degree to which he can function independently.

The following are some of the ways in which physicians and therapists utilize the evaluation of joint motion as part of a patient's permanent record: (1) An accurate record of joint motion provides information which is necessary for determining the extent of disability. It is important for the establishment of realistic goals, including an estimate of the degree of rehabilitation that is feasible for the patient. (2) The joint measurement record will indicate those treatment procedures required to improve the functional ability of the patient. It will also provide a basis for establishing the appropriate activity level for the patient — the activities which he should be capable of and should be expected to perform at any given time. (3) Periodic measurements, properly recorded, provide a means of objectively evaluating progress of the patient and provide data for evaluating the effectiveness of the treatment regime. They may also be an important factor in the motivation of the patient. (4) Only through research can the value of a therapeutic procedure be scientifically assessed. If accurate and comparable measurements are available, they can become the foundation of meaningful studies.

The most common methods of evaluating joint measurement employ the goniometer as the measuring instrument. Directions for the two most common systems of recording the results of the measurement, the 180° system and the 360° system, will be included in this manual. In describing motion quantitatively, both systems depend on the fact that a long bone is like a lever rotating around a fulcrum. As it moves it describes the arc of a circle. This arc is used to determine the amount of motion which has occurred.

Although normal joint mobility allows a wide variety of motions, standardization of the measurement method requires specific definitions of each motion to be evaluated. For this reason, movement as it occurs around an axis perpendicular to one of the three body planes, sagittal, coronal, or transverse, is measured. See Figure 1. In the following list of motions asterisks designate those which, in the 360° system, are not related to the full circle; an arbitrary starting position has been designated and these motions are calculated as deviations from 0°.

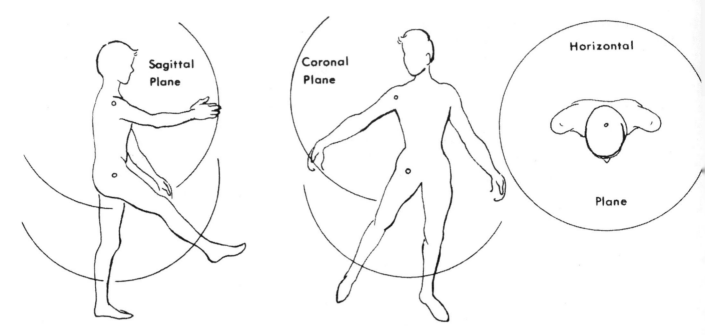

Figure 1. Planes of motion

Place the point of a toothpick on either dot. It represents the coronal axis. The arm and thigh flex and extend in a sagittal plane.

Holding the toothpick on one of these dots demonstrates the sagittal axis. Abduction and adduction occur in the coronal plane.

In this example the toothpick represents the vertical axis. Rotation of the head, arm, leg, or trunk occurs in the horizontal plane.

Motions in a Sagittal Plane around a Coronal Axis

> Shoulder: Flexion and extension. Internal and external rotation.
> Elbow: Flexion and extension
> Wrist: Flexion and extension
> Fingers: Flexion and extension
> Hip: Flexion and extension
> Knee: Flexion and extension
> Ankle: Dorsi and plantar flexion
> Thumb: *Abduction

Motions in a Coronal Plane around a Sagittal Axis

> Shoulder: Abduction and adduction
> Wrist: *Radial and ulnar deviation
> Thumb: *Extension
> Hip: Abduction and adduction
> Foot: *Eversion and inversion

Forearm: *Supination and pronation
Hip: *Internal and external rotation

Figure 2 demonstrates motion at the elbow joint. As the forearm moves, the hand describes the arc of a circle. To provide a numerical system for analysis of motion a 0° position of the circle is arbitrarily designated. In Figure 2 the 0° position is designated at the position of maximum elbow extension, which is the anatomic position, and the hand describes a 150° arc of motion as it moves to maximal flexion.

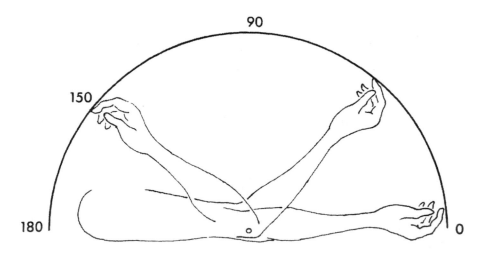

Figure 2. Motion at the elbow joint

The goniometer is used to measure the angle produced between two bony segments when maximal motion in a particular plane is achieved. It is a simple device with two levers, or arms, and with a protractor attached at the end of one arm. See Figure 5. The other arm forms a pointer at the end. At the center of the protractor, where the two arms join, an axis allows movement. The goniometer is placed on the extremity with its axis centered on the joint and its arms aligned with designated skeletal landmarks. For elbow flexion and extension, as shown in Figure 2, one arm of the goniometer would be aligned with the humerus and the other with the radius. The axis would be located at the elbow joint. The reading on the protractor scale for extension would be 0° and the reading for flexion would be 150°. The forearm has moved in a sagittal plane from extension to flexion resulting in a total range of motion of 150°.

Assessment of disability in a patient requires that the results of joint measurement on him be compared with a norm. If the patient has a unilateral disability the measurements of his unaffected extremity should be used for comparison. Measurements may also be compared to an established normal range of motion. In this manual you will find the normal limits given for each motion. These are only _averages_ which were calculated following the measurement of a number of normal subjects. Slight variations are found in the normal limits given by various authorities. Consequently, it must be remembered that they are not absolute figures and can only be used as a guide for what may be normal for any individual. Also to be considered are a number of nonpathological factors which may affect normal joint mobility, some of which are the following: (1) hereditary and constitutional factors; (2) sex; (3) age; (4) physical training and activity; (5) occupation; (6) posture; (7) anxiety or stress.

THE 180° SYSTEM

For the 180° system the 0° position is designated as the starting position of each motion. In most instances the starting position is comparable to the anatomic position and the half circle should be visualized as superimposed on the body in the plane in which motion will occur. The 180° position is directly overhead and the 0° position toward the feet. All motions are from 0° toward 180°.

The motions at the wrist and shoulder in the sagittal plane are different from all others — motion is possible in both directions from the 0° anatomic position. The term _hyperextension_ is used to describe motion in a posterior direction from the starting position.

Figure 3 shows the normal range of motion of the shoulder in flexion and extension. Shoulder flexion would be recorded as 170° and hyperextension as 60°. The total range of motion is 230° — 170° plus 60°.

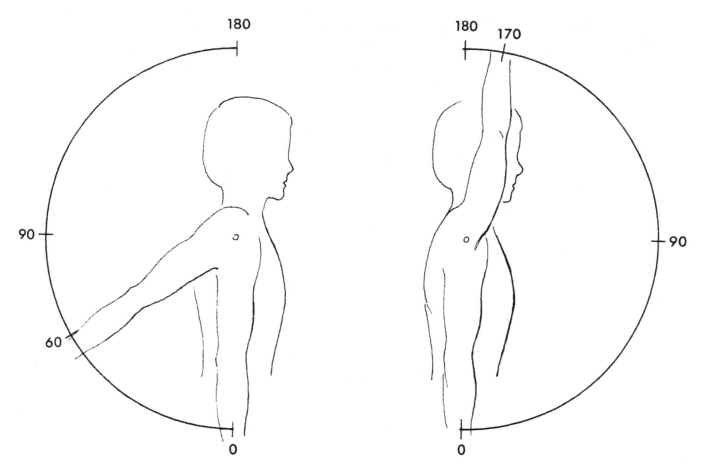

Figure 3. Motion of the shoulder in flexion and extension (180° system)

THE 360° SYSTEM

The 360° system relates movements occurring in the coronal and sagittal planes to a full circle. With the body in anatomic position, the circle may be visualized as superimposed on it in the same plane in which motion will occur. The 0° (360°) position will be overhead and the 180° position toward the feet. Thus flexion and abduction are motions toward 0° and adduction and extension are toward 360°.

Certain motions (see page 5) cannot be related to the full circle for measurement. For these motions a starting position is arbitrarily designated and they are measured as deviations from 0°.

Figure 4 shows the normal range of motion of the shoulder in flexion and extension. Shoulder flexion would be recorded as 10° and extension as 240°. The total range of motion is then 230° — 240° minus 10°.

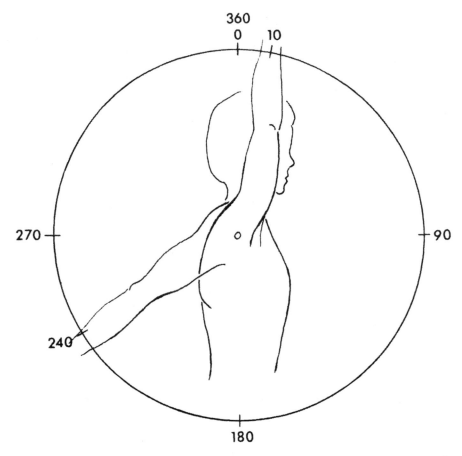

Figure 4. Range of motion of the shoulder in flexion and extension (360° system)

GONIOMETERS

Goniometers are generally made of plastic or metal and are available from a number of hospital equipment supply companies. They vary in size from small pocket models to rather large ones. The advantage of the small goniometer is that it may be carried in the pocket, which is convenient if you are seeing ward patients. The small goniometer is also more satisfactory for measuring the smaller joints such as the fingers. The advantage of the goniometer with longer arms is its greater accuracy in measuring the larger joints such as the hip: the longer arms can be lined up with the body segments with more accuracy.

Goniometers are either 180° (half circle) or 360° (full circle). The full-circle goniometer is somewhat more convenient to use with the 360° system because it has the complete circle scale and readings in excess of 180° may be taken directly from the scale. Half-circle goniometers pose no real problem in measuring; one can adapt to their use with relative ease. Their inconvenience lies in the fact that you must add degrees if an extremity moves beyond 180° and also that it must be reversed in some cases resulting in the scale facing the body of your subject. The goniometer must then be removed from your subject's body and reversed so that the scale may be read.

One very important feature to look for on a goniometer is a locking nut for the fulcrum. The locking nut is tightened just before removing the goniometer from the body segment, assuring an accurate reading. See Figure 5.

There are other types of goniometers on the market. Some incorporate fluids with a free floating bubble. The bubble provides the reading upon completion of motion.

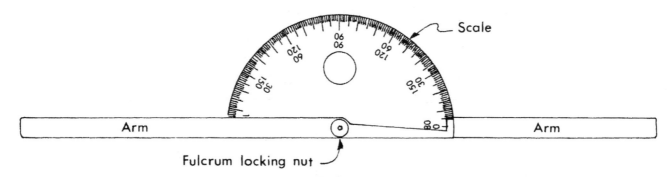

180° (half-circle) goniometer in starting position

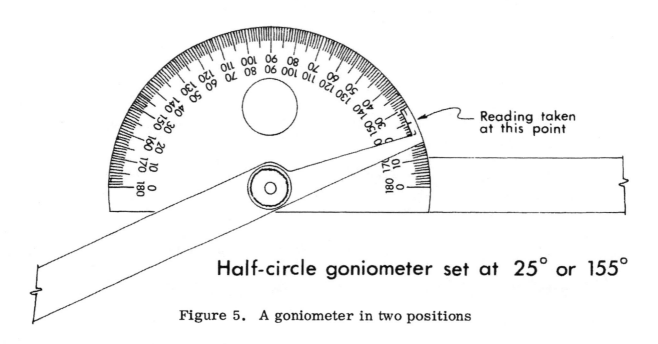

Half-circle goniometer set at 25° or 155°

Figure 5. A goniometer in two positions

General Procedures

The following are the general procedures recommended for measurement of joint motion.

1. Evaluation of the patient should be done in a room which is warm and well lighted. The measurement process and its purpose should be explained. During the evaluation you should be alert to signs of discomfort or fatigue. Requiring your subject to maintain a given position for a prolonged period will cause muscle fatigue which may result in decreased motion.

2. Expose the extremity to be measured using draping when appropriate.

3. Place the extremity in the proper testing position. For teaching purposes this manual has specified testing positions. Actually positions vary but should allow freedom of movement and attempt to decrease the probability of compensatory motion. As previously indicated, the calculation of range of motion (ROM) is based on movement which starts with the extremity in anatomic position or an arbitrary starting position. The preferred testing positions do not always exactly duplicate anatomic position. For purposes of calculation it will be necessary for you to visualize the circle superimposed on the extremity with the 0° position placed as it would be if the extremity were in anatomic position. Figures 6 and 7 demonstrate this process.

4. Instruct your subject to move the extremity through the desired range of motion. Be sure that the extremity is maintained in the proper plane of motion since deviations will result in inaccurate measurement.

5. When maximum motion is achieved the measurement should be taken, using the goniometer as follows:

The fulcrum must be centered over the joint and the arms lined up properly on the body segments. Readings should be taken as quickly as possible to minimize fatiguing of the patient.

The preferred method of taking a reading is to have your patient complete the range, watch for substitutions, and then line up the goniometer for measurement.

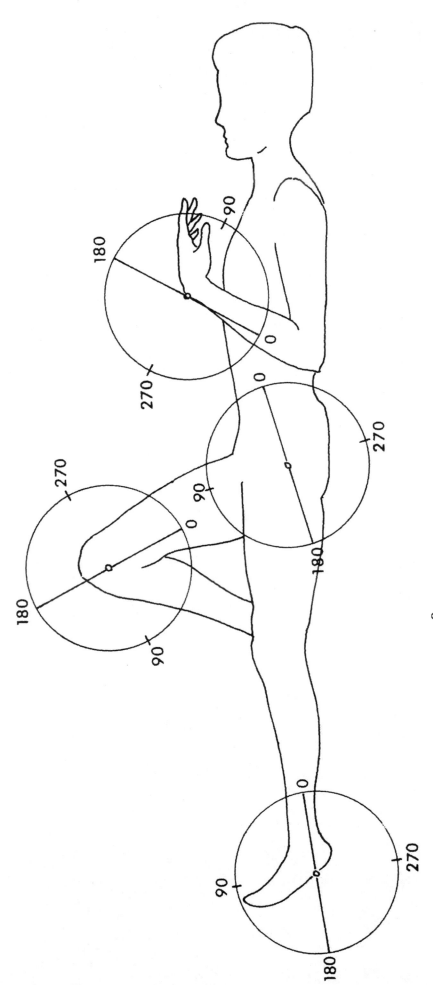

Figure 6. The 360° system. Regardless of the testing position, the 0° position of the circle must be located as it would be if the extremity were in anatomic position.

11

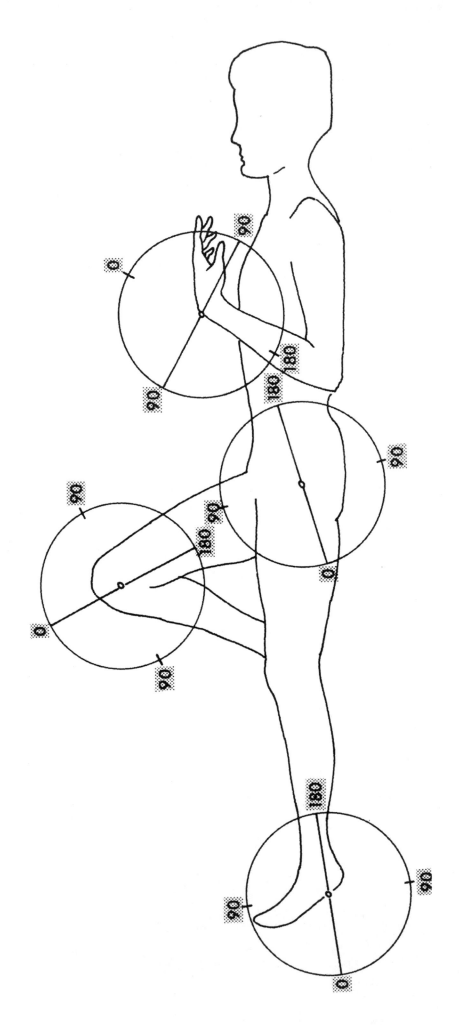

Figure 7. The 180° system. Regardless of the testing position the 0° position must be located as it would be if the extremity were in anatomic position.

Metal goniometers should be pre-warmed with your hands before placing them in contact with the patient's skin. In addition, you must be careful not to pinch the patient's skin or catch hair between the arm and the scale as you use the goniometer. It is frequently unnecessary to hold the goniometer in direct contact with the skin. It can be held a short distance away without loss of accuracy. Your eyes should be in a direct line with the scale. Reading a goniometer at an angle results in inaccurate reading. The goniometer should be carefully placed: fulcrum over the axis of the joint and the arms centered along the body segments. See Figure 8. The eye of the person reading the goniometer should be on a level with the scale to assure accuracy.

6. The measurement may be of passive or active motion and this should be specified on the record. For various reasons these may vary and in many instances both active and passive motion should be measured.

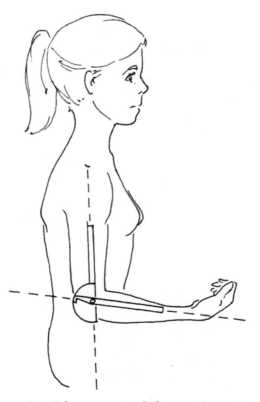

Figure 8. Placement of the goniometer

Upper Extremity Measurement and Recording

The following study method is recommended:

1. In the classroom setting it is recommended that subjects being measured complete less than normal limits of motion. Doing this will produce a more realistic experience, more similar to measuring an extremity with actual joint limitation.

2. Study each illustration noting goniometer placement and the normal limits of motion.

3. Read the instructions for testing position and goniometer placement.

4. Place your subject in the proper testing position as described. Have him complete the range of motion he is capable of producing.

5. Place the goniometer as directed and carefully take a reading.

6. Enter the readings in the spaces provided. Calculate the total range of motion (ROM) and enter the figure in the space provided.

Shoulder Flexion and Extension

TESTING POSITION: Arm at side.   Forearm extended.   Palm facing body.

GONIOMETER PLACEMENT:
Fulcrum: Center at the shoulder joint just below the acromion.
Arms: (1) Parallel to the mid-axillary line of the trunk.   (2) Parallel to
   the longitudinal axis of the humerus along the lateral side.

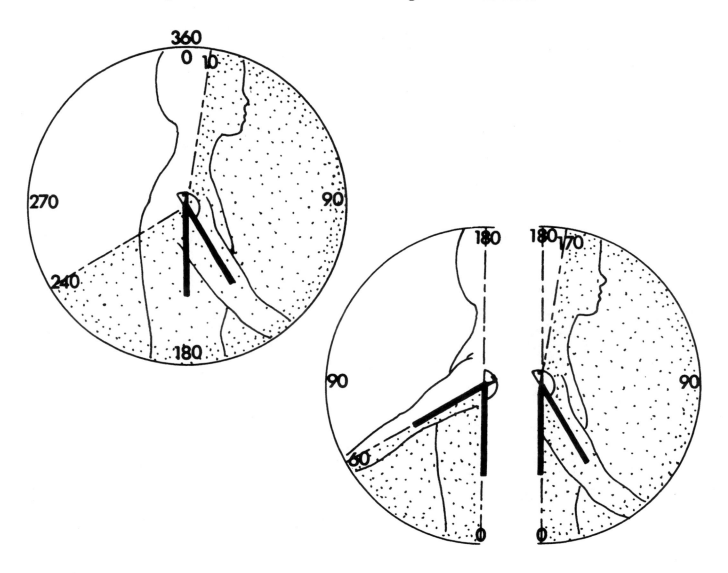

<u>Joint Measurement Record</u>:

(180° System) Flexion_____ Hyperextension_____ Total ROM _____.
(360° System) Flexion_____ Extension _____ Total ROM_____.

Shoulder Abduction and Adduction

TESTING POSITION: Arm at side. Forearm extended. Palm facing body.

GONIOMETER PLACEMENT:
Fulcrum: Center at the shoulder joint, posteriorly.
Arms: (1) Parallel with the midline of the body. (Longitudinal axis of the
vertebral column.) (2) Parallel to the longitudinal axis of the humerus.

Note: It is necessary to rotate externally at the end of the range to
achieve maximum abduction.

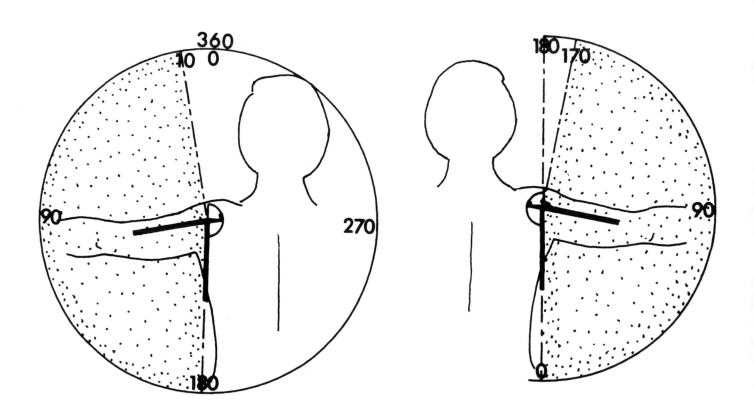

Joint Measurement Record:

(180° System) Abduction_____ Adduction_____ Total ROM_____.
(360° System) Abduction_____ Adduction_____ Total ROM_____.

Shoulder Rotation

TESTING POSITION: Arm abducted to 90°.   Elbow flexed to 90°.   Palm down.

GONIOMETER PLACEMENT:
Fulcrum: Center on the elbow joint.
Arms: (1) Parallel to the mid-axillary line of the thorax.   (2) Parallel to the longitudinal axis of the ulna.

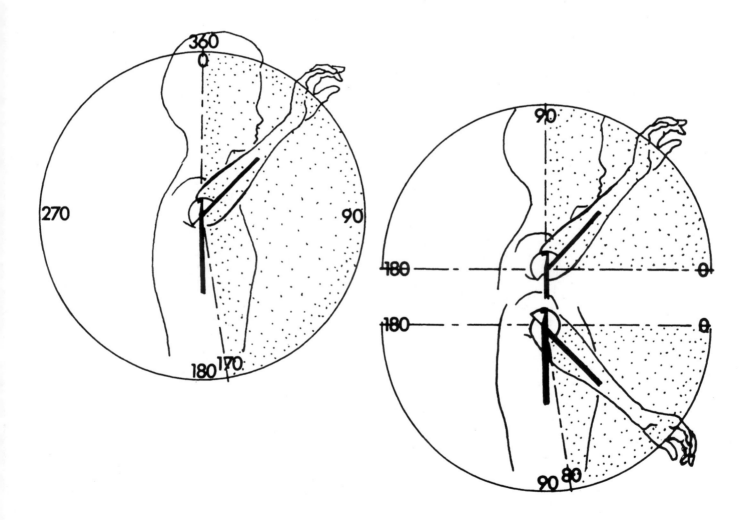

Joint Measurement Record:

(180° System) Int. Rotation_____Ext. Rotation_____Total ROM____.
(360° System) Int. Rotation_____Ext. Rotation_____Total ROM____.

Elbow Flexion and Extension

TESTING POSITION: Arm at side. Forearm extended and supinated.

GONIOMETER PLACEMENT:
Fulcrum: Centered over lateral aspect of the elbow joint.
Arms: (1) Parallel to the longitudinal axis of the humerus. (2) Parallel to the longitudinal axis of the radius.

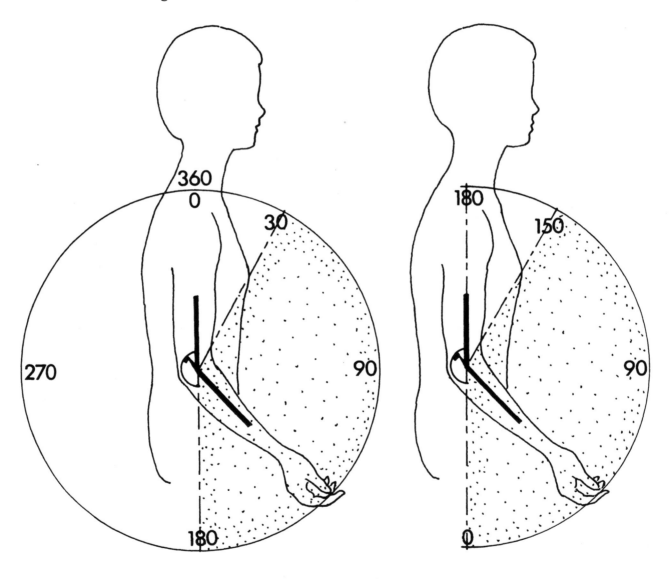

Joint Measurement Record:

(180° System) Flexion_____ Extension_____ Total ROM_____.
(360° System) Flexion_____ Extension_____ Total ROM_____.

Pronation and Supination

TESTING POSITION: Arm adducted, elbow flexed to 90°, to rule out
shoulder rotation. Forearm midway between pronation and supination.

GONIOMETER PLACEMENT:
Fulcrum: Centered at the ulnar styloid.
Arms: (1) Parallel with the longitudinal axis of the humerus anteriorly.
(2) Pronation — on the dorsal surface of the wrist. Supination — on
the volar surface of the wrist.

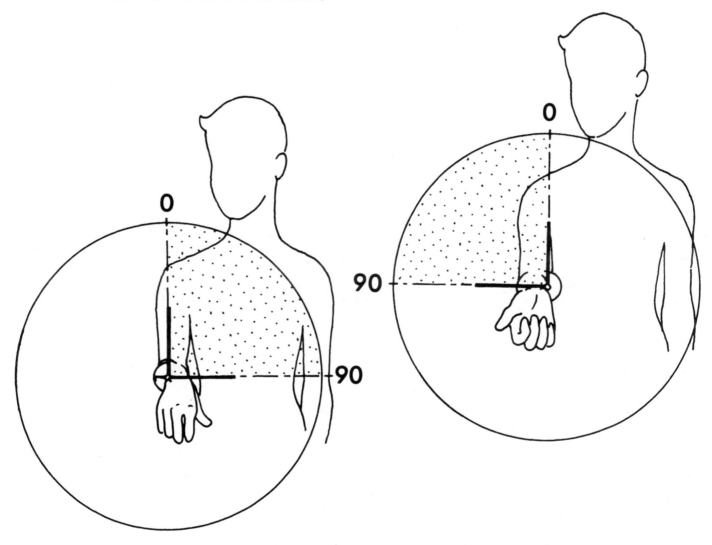

Joint Measurement Record:

(Both Systems) Pronation_____Supination_____Total ROM_____.

Wrist Flexion and Extension

TESTING POSITION: Arm at side. Elbow flexed to a comfortable position.
Palm down.

GONIOMETER PLACEMENT:
Fulcrum: Centered at the ulnar styloid.
Arms: (1) Parallel to the longitudinal axis of the ulna. (2) Parallel to
the longitudinal axis of the fifth metacarpal.

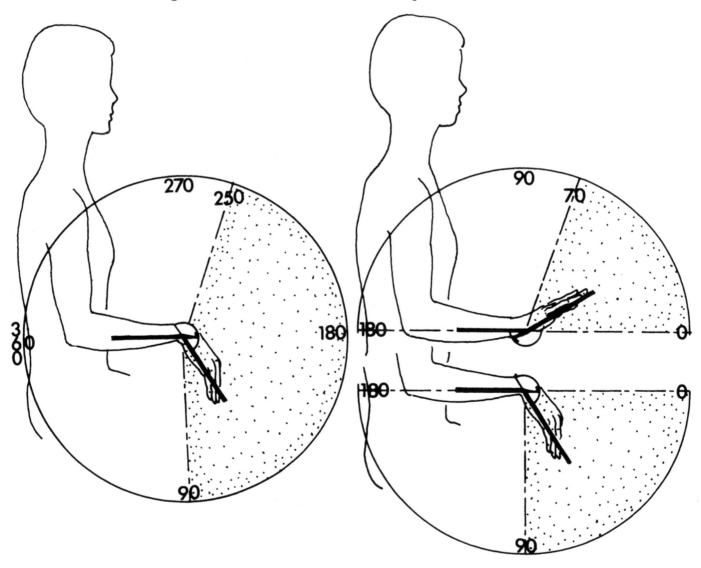

Joint Measurement Record:

(180° System) Flexion _____ Extension _____ Total ROM _____.
(360° System) Flexion _____ Extension _____ Total ROM _____.

Radial and Ulnar Deviation

TESTING POSITION: Arm at side. Elbow flexed to a comfortable position. Forearm pronated.

GONIOMETER PLACEMENT:
Fulcrum: Centered just proximal to the third metacarpal over the capitate.
Arms: (1) Along the midline of the dorsal surface of the forearm.
    (2) Parallel to the longitudinal axis of the third metacarpal.

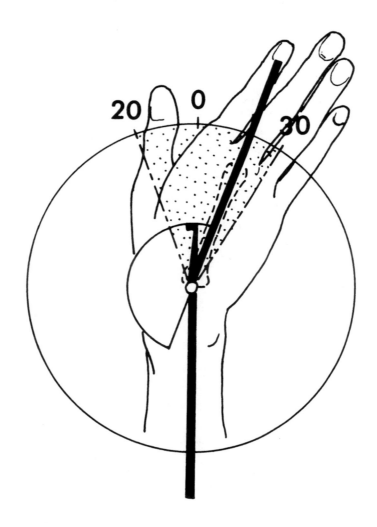

Joint Measurement Record:

(Both Systems) Radial Dev._____Ulnar Dev._____Total ROM_____.

Metacarpophalangeal Flexion and Extension

TESTING POSITION: Hand in a comfortable position for measurement. Wrist in a neutral position as illustrated to allow for proper placement of the goniometer.

GONIOMETER:

Fulcrum: Centered at the metacarpophalangeal joint.

Arms: (1) On the dorsum of the metacarpal. (2) On the dorsum of the proximal phalanx.

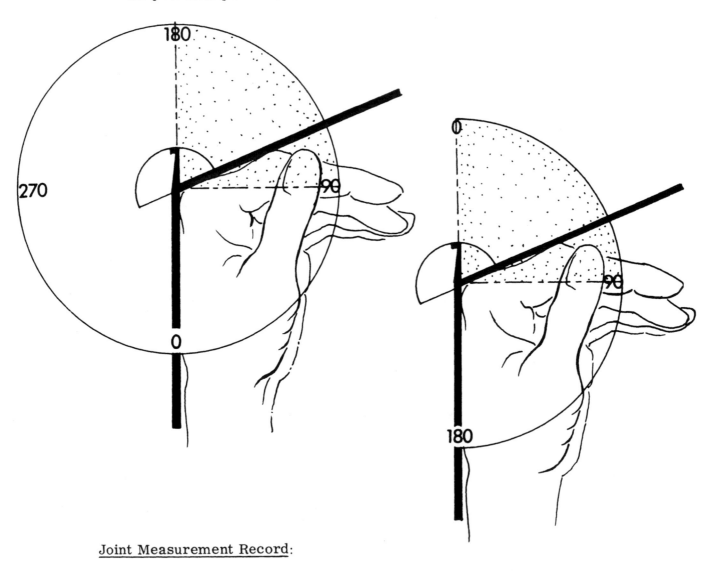

Joint Measurement Record:

(180° System) Flexion_____ Extension_____Total ROM_____.
(360° System) Flexion_____ Extension_____Total ROM_____.

Proximal Interphalangeal Flexion and Extension

TESTING POSITION: Hand in a comfortable position for measurement. Wrist in a neutral or slightly dorsiflexed position.

GONIOMETER PLACEMENT:
Fulcrum: Centered at the proximal interphalangeal joint.
Arms: (1) On the dorsal surface of the proximal phalanx. (2) On the dorsal surface of the middle phalanx.

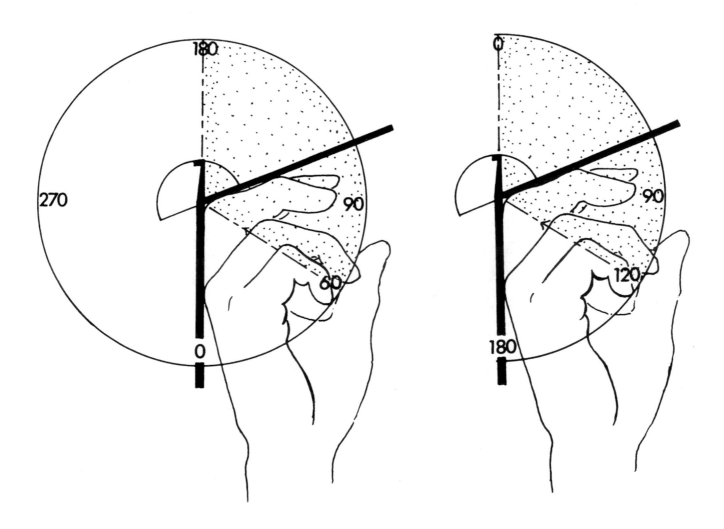

Joint Measurement Record:

    (180º System) Flexion_____ Extension_____Total ROM_____.
    (360º System) Flexion_____ Extension_____Total ROM_____.

Distal Interphalangeal Flexion and Extension

TESTING POSITION: Hand in a comfortable position for measurement. Wrist in a neutral or slightly dorsiflexed position.

GONIOMETER PLACEMENT:
Fulcrum: Centered at the distal interphalangeal joint.
Arms: (1) On the dorsal surface of the middle phalanx. (2) On the dorsal surface of the distal phalanx.

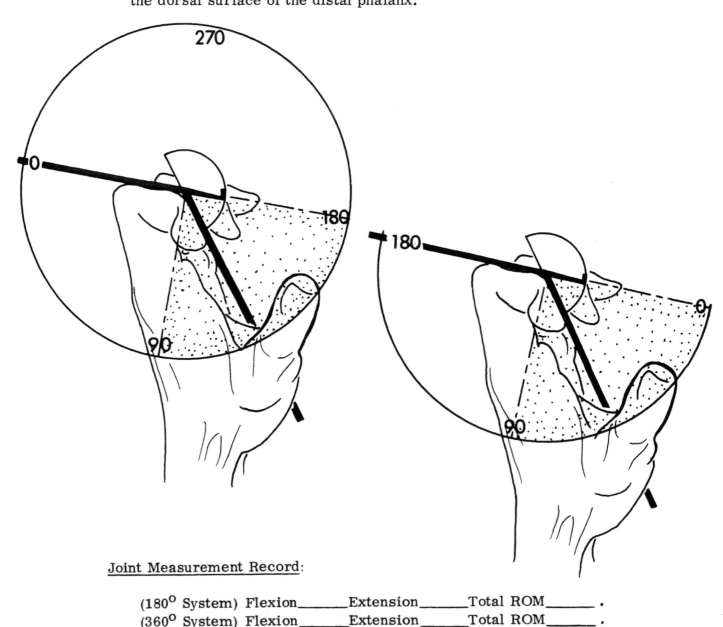

Joint Measurement Record:

(180° System) Flexion_____Extension_____Total ROM_____.
(360° System) Flexion_____Extension_____Total ROM_____.

Thumb Carpometacarpal Extension

TESTING POSITION: Hand supinated.

GONIOMETER PLACEMENT:
Arms: (1) Along the volar surface of the third metacarpal. (2) Parallel to the midline of the first metacarpal.

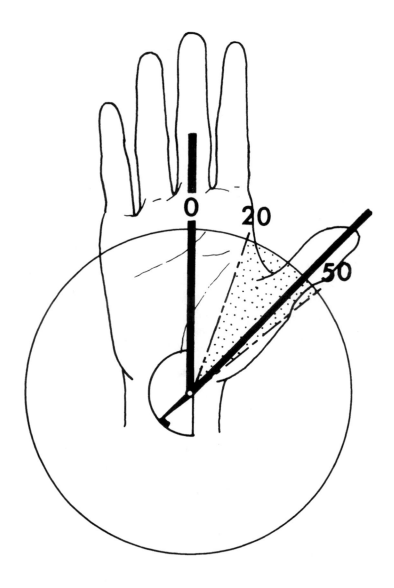

Joint Measurement Record:

(Both Systems) Extension from ___ to ___ Total ROM _____ .

Thumb Metacarpophalangeal Flexion and Extension

TESTING POSITION: Hand supinated.

GONIOMETER PLACEMENT:
Fulcrum: Centered at the metacarpophalangeal joint.
Arms: (1) On the dorsal surface of the first metacarpal. (2) On the dorsal surface of the proximal phalanx.

Note: Mobility of the metacarpophalangeal joint of the thumb varies. It should fall within the limits specified.

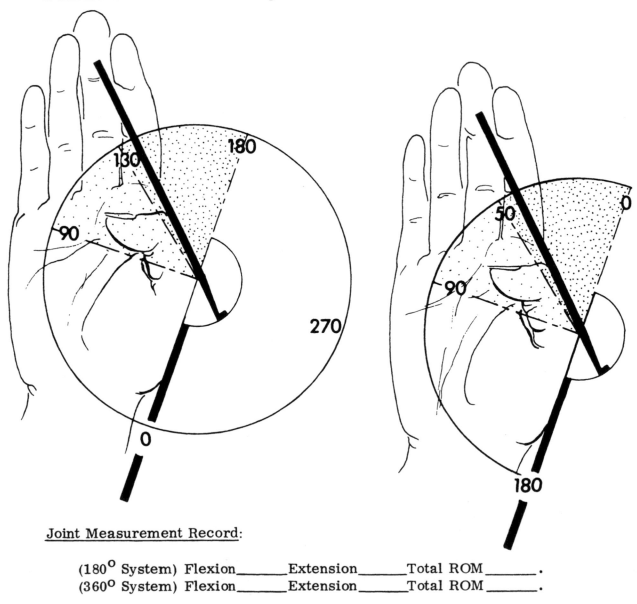

Joint Measurement Record:

(180° System) Flexion_____Extension_____Total ROM_____.
(360° System) Flexion_____Extension_____Total ROM_____.

Thumb Interphalangeal Flexion and Extension

TESTING POSITION: Hand supinated.

GONIOMETER PLACEMENT:
Fulcrum: Centered at the interphalangeal joint.
Arms: (1) On the dorsal surface of the proximal phalanx. (2) On the dorsal surface of the distal phalanx.

Note: Thumb interphalangeal flexion and extension vary. Flexion should approximate 90° as illustrated.

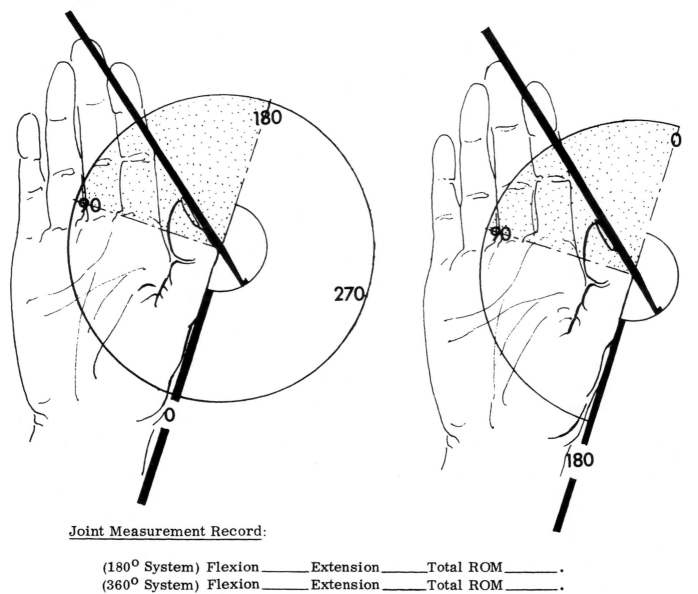

Joint Measurement Record:

(180° System) Flexion_____Extension_____Total ROM_____.
(360° System) Flexion_____Extension_____Total ROM_____.

Abduction of Thumb

TESTING POSITION: Forearm midway between pronation and supination.

GONIOMETER PLACEMENT:
Arms: (1) Along the lateral surface of the second metacarpal. (2) Parallel to the midline of the first metacarpal.

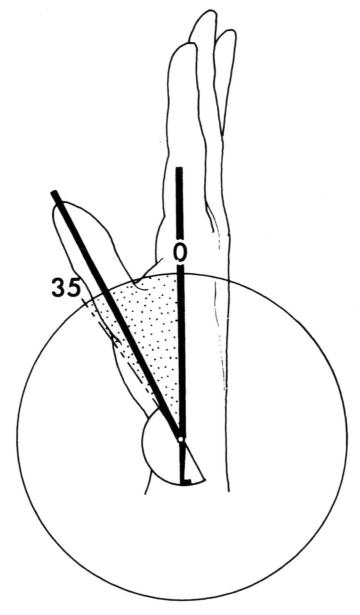

Joint Measurement Record:

(Both Systems) Adduction_____Abduction_____Total ROM_____.

Optional Method: Fingers and Thumb (Graphic Representation)

Graphic representation is an evaluative procedure which may be substituted for or supplemental to goniometric measurement of the fingers and thumb. Because it results in a picture, it may be more meaningful to the patient and may help to increase motivation. Graphic representation may also be useful to health care team members unfamiliar with goniometry. It may be used for flexion, extension, abduction, and adduction of the fingers and thumb. The procedure is as follows.

Abduction and Adduction

1.   Draw a straight line through the center of an 8 1/2" x 11" sheet of paper.

2.   Place the hand, palm down, on the paper, with the third finger centered over the line.

3.   Draw around each finger and the thumb in the adducted position.

4.   Ask your subject to abduct the fingers and thumb and draw around them again. In order to represent abduction of the third finger it should be moved first in a radial direction and then in an ulnar direction.

5.   The patient's name and hospital number, the therapist's name, the type of motion (passive or active), and the date should be recorded on each drawing. Left or right hand should be specified.

6.   The drawings should be repeated on separate sheets, generally once a week, to record progress or regression. The sheets may be overlayed and held up to a light source to illustrate change in motion. It is possible to record both abduction and adduction on a single sheet; however, the overlay of lines becomes confusing.

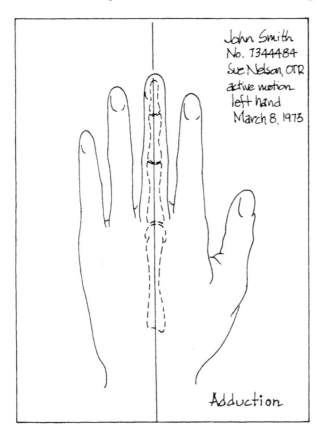

John Smith
No. 7344484
Sue Nelson, OTR
active motion
left hand
March 8, 1973

Adduction

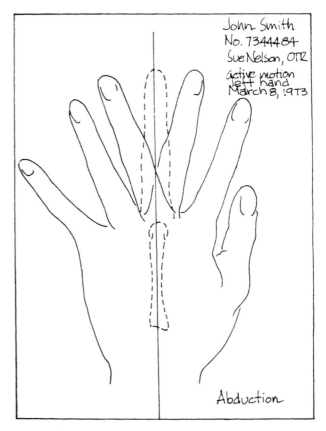

John Smith
No. 7344484
Sue Nelson, OTR
active motion
left hand
March 8, 1973

Abduction

The third metacarpal should be maintained over the center line as the fingers are moved.

The middle finger should be abducted ulnarward and radial-ward from the center line.

Flexion and Extension

1. Place the ulnar side of the index finger on the edge of a 5" x 8" file card. <u>The card will be at right angles to the dorsal surface of the hand.</u>

2. With the metacarpophalangeal and interphalangeal joints in maximal extension, draw around the finger.

3. Ask your subject to flex his finger and draw around it in this position.

4. Progress will be shown best if the periodic drawings are done on the same sheet or cards. The use of a different colored pencil for each drawing is recommended.

5. Record the same information on each card as was necessary for abduction and adduction.

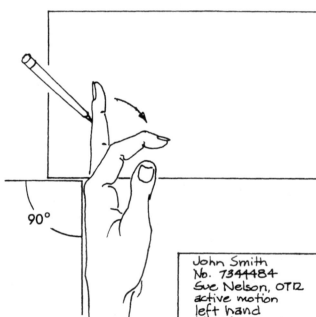

90°

Maintain a 90° angle between the dorsum of the hand and the card. Trace around the finger in the fully extended position and then in maximal flexion.

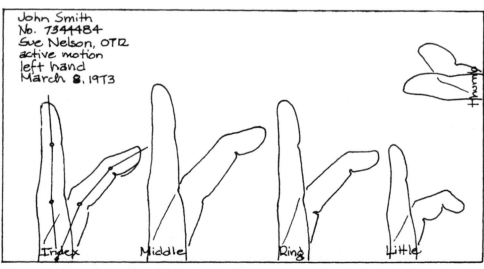

John Smith
No. 7344484
Sue Nelson, OTR
active motion
left hand
March 8, 1973

Index   Middle   Ring   Little   thumb

The illustration shows a completed card. Lines may be projected along the center line of each finger and the joint axis indicated if desired. A goniometer can then be superimposed on the line and axis to record degrees of motion.

Lower Extremity Measurement and Recording

Follow the recommended study methods outlined for the upper extremities.

Hip Flexion and Extension

TESTING POSITION: For flexion - supine; for extension - prone.

GONIOMETER PLACEMENT:
Fulcrum: Centered at the greater trochanter.
Arms: (1) Draw a line from the anterior superior iliac spine (ASIS) to the posterior superior iliac spine (PSIS). Drop a perpendicular line from this line through the greater trochanter. Place one arm of the goniometer on this perpendicular line. (2) Parallel to the longitudinal axis of the femur.

Note: Positioning for hip extension is not illustrated. For extension the subject is placed in a prone position. Normal limits for extension are provided in the illustrations below. (See the next page for an alternate method of hip measurement.)

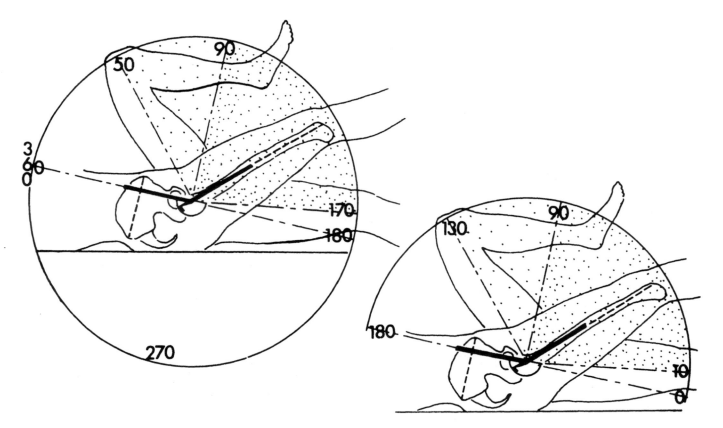

Joint Measurement Record:

(180° System) Flexion_____ Extension_____ Total ROM_____.
(360° System) Flexion_____ Extension_____ Total ROM_____.

Alternate Method:
Hip Flexion and Extension

This method of measurement is subject to inaccuracy because of posterior pelvic tilt. As the leg extends so does the lumbar spine. Therefore, one must be as careful as possible that motion is confined to the hip joint. This is, however, almost impossible to achieve. The result is a greater excursion of extension, part of it hip joint, part of it lumbar spine.

TESTING POSITION: For flexion - supine; for extension - prone.

GONIOMETER PLACEMENT:
Fulcrum: Centered at the greater trochanter.
Arms: (1) Parallel to the longitudinal axis of the trunk. (2) Parallel to the longitudinal axis of the femur.

Note: Only measurement of extension is illustrated. For flexion your subject is supine and the goniometer placement is the same as for extension. Maximal limits for flexion with knee extended using the 180° system are 90° and for the 360° system 90°. With the knee flexed, 180° system 130° and 360° system 50°.

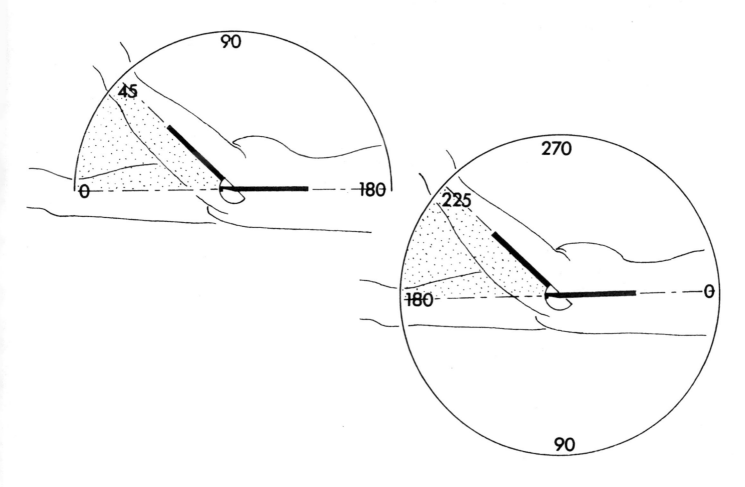

Joint Measurement Record:

(180° System) Flexion_____ Extension_____ Total ROM_____.
(360° System) Flexion_____ Extension_____ Total ROM_____.

Hip Abduction and Adduction

GONIOMETER PLACEMENT:

Arms: (1) Parallel to a line drawn between the two anterior superior
iliac spines - at the level of the greater trochanter. (An alternate
method places the goniometer on the line between the two anterior
superior iliac spines.) (2) Parallel to the longitudinal axis of the
femur.

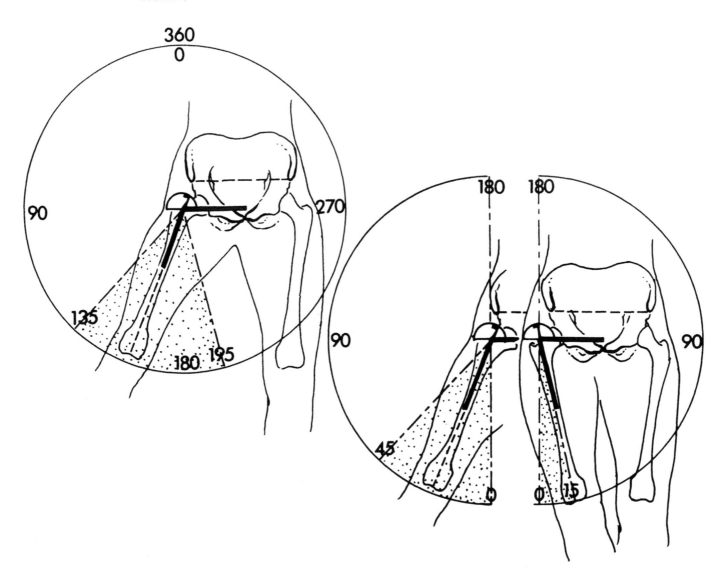

Joint Measurement Record:

(180° System) Adduction_____ Abduction_____ Total ROM_____.
(360° System) Adduction_____ Abduction_____ Total ROM_____.

Hip External and Internal Rotation

TESTING POSITION: (1) Sitting with the knee flexed to 90°. (2) Supine
    with the knee flexed to 90°.

GONIOMETER PLACEMENT:

Fulcrum: Centered on the anterior surface of the knee joint.

Arms: Both arms are placed parallel to the longitudinal axis of the
    tibia with the leg in the testing position. One arm remains in
    this position and the other follows the tibia as the hip is rotated.

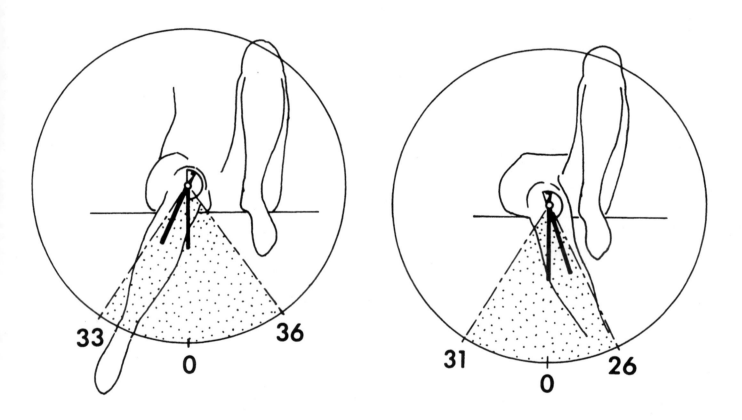

<u>Joint Measurement Record</u>:

    (Both Systems) Ext. Rotation____ Int. Rotation____Total ROM_____ .

Knee Flexion and Extension

GONIOMETER PLACEMENT:
Fulcrum: Centered on the lateral side of the knee joint.
Arms: (1) Parallel to the longitudinal axis of the femur. (2) Parallel
to the longitudinal axis of the tibia.

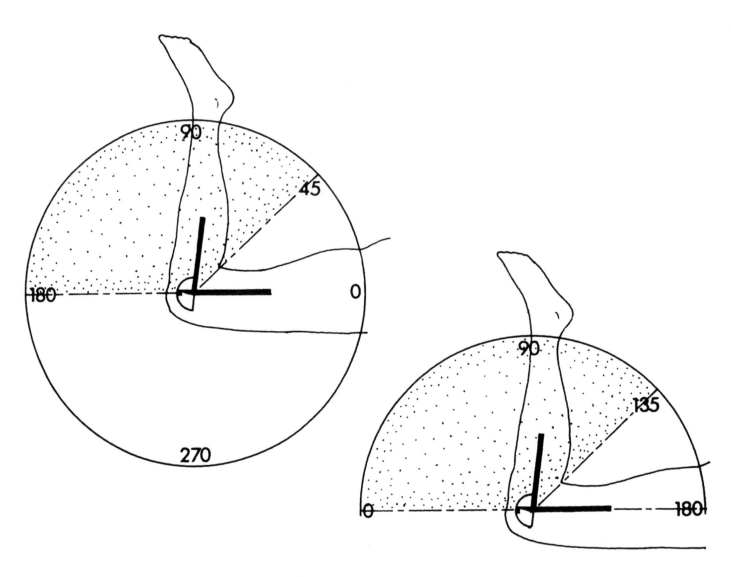

Joint Measurement Record:

(180° System) Flexion_____ Extension_____Total ROM_____ .
(360° System) Flexion_____ Extension_____Total ROM_____ .

Dorsiflexion and Plantar Flexion

TESTING POSITION: Sitting with the knee flexed.

GONIOMETER PLACEMENT:

Fulcrum: Center at the sole of the foot in line with the longitudinal axis of the fibula.

Arms: (1) Parallel to the longitudinal axis of the fibula. (2) Parallel to the longitudinal axis of the fifth metatarsal.

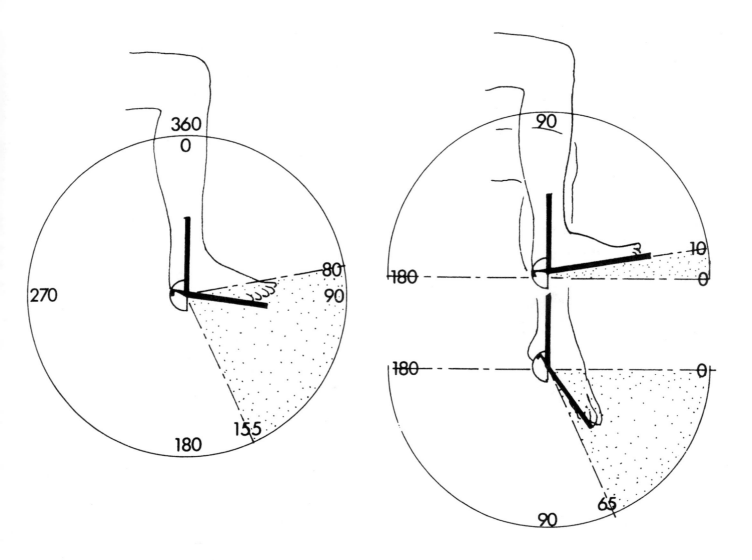

Joint Measurement Record:

(180° System) Plantar Flex_____ Dorsiflex_____ Total ROM_____.
(360° System) Plantar Flex_____ Dorsiflex_____ Total ROM_____.

Inversion and Eversion

TESTING POSITION: Sitting with the knee flexed.

GONIOMETER PLACEMENT:
Arms: Eversion (1) Parallel to the longitudinal axis of the tibia medially.
(2) Parallel to the plantar surface of the sole. Inversion (1) Parallel
to the longitudinal axis of the tibia laterally. (2) Parallel to the
plantar surface of the heel.

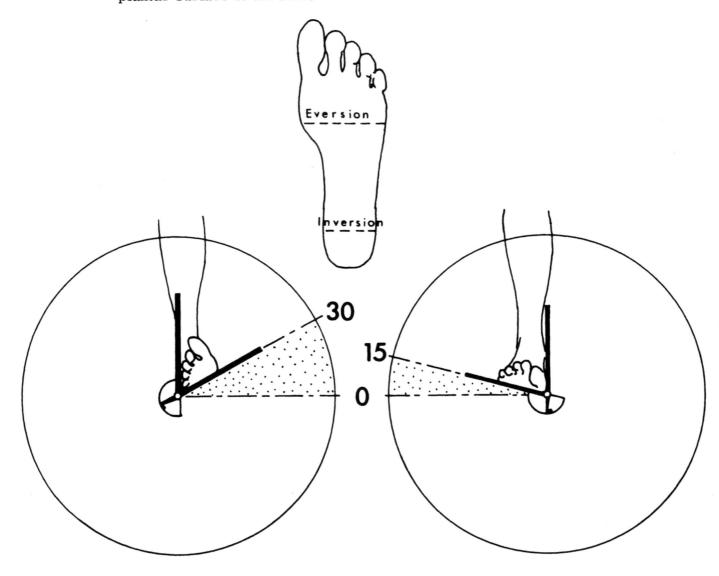

Joint Measurement Record:

(Both Systems) Inversion_____Eversion_____Total ROM_____.

REFERENCES AND INDEX

References

Clayson SJ, Mundale MO, Kottke FJ: Goniometer Adaptation for
Measuring Hip Extension. Arch Phys Med 47: 255, 1966.

Joint Motion: A Method of Measuring and Recording. Chicago,
American Academy of Orthopaedic Surgeons, 1965.

Moore ML in Licht: Therapeutic Exercise, 2nd ed. revised. New
Haven, Elizabeth Licht, Publisher, 1965, pp. 128-162.

Muscle Function Tests and Measurements, Laboratory Manual.
Course in Physical Therapy, University of Minnesota.

Index